Meatless Lean & Green Air Fryer Recipes

A Complete Cookbook Full of Yummy Meatless Dishes

Roxana Sutton

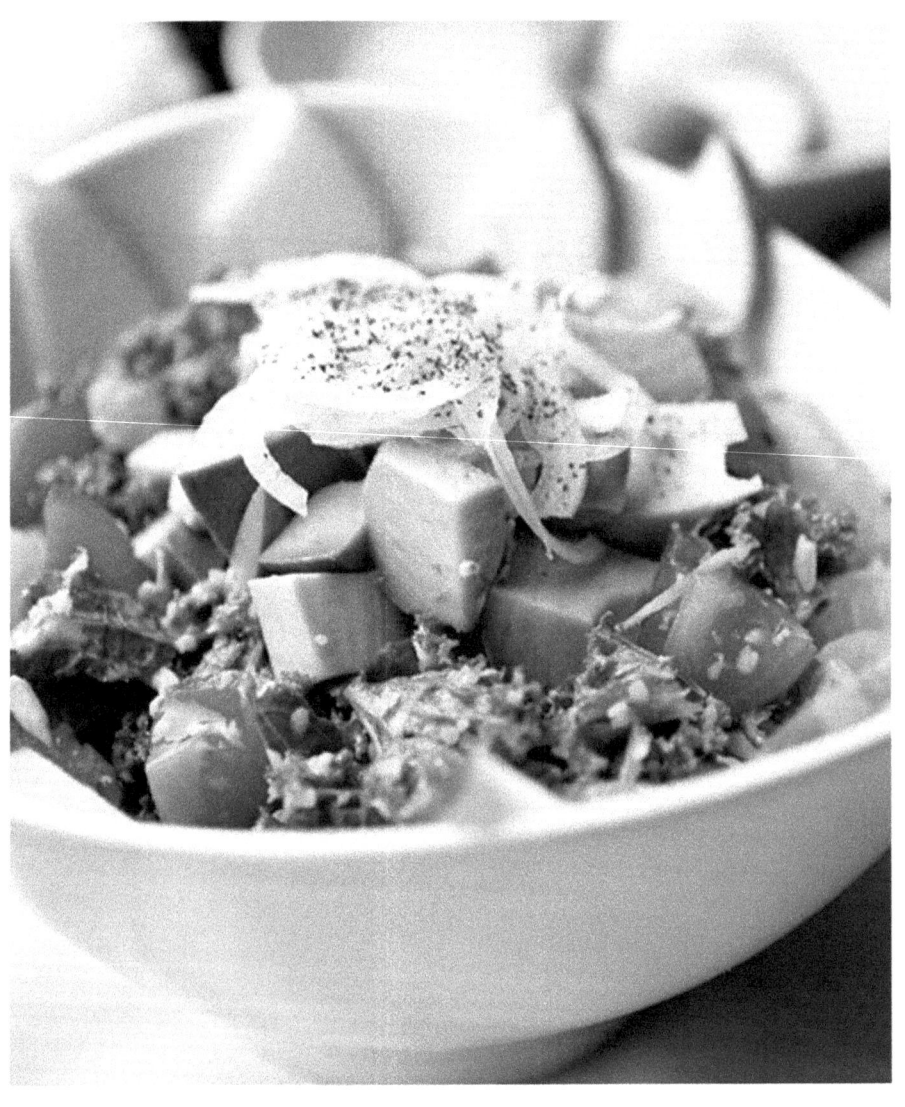

© Copyright 2021 - All rights reserved.

The content contained within this book may not be reproduced, duplicated or transmitted without direct written permission from the author or the publisher.
Under no circumstances will any blame or legal responsibility be held against the publisher, or author, for any damages, reparation, or monetary loss due to the information contained within this book. Either directly or indirectly.

Legal Notice:

This book is copyright protected. This book is only for personal use. You cannot amend, distribute, sell, use, quote or paraphrase any part, or the content within this book, without the consent of the author or publisher.

Disclaimer Notice:

Please note the information contained within this document is for educational and entertainment purposes only. All effort has been executed to present accurate, up to date, and reliable, complete information. No warranties of any kind are declared or implied. Readers acknowledge that the author is not engaging in the rendering of legal, financial, medical or professional advice. The content within this book has been derived from various sources. Please consult a licensed professional before attempting any techniques outlined in this book.

By reading this document, the reader agrees that under no circumstances is the author responsible for any losses, direct or indirect, which are incurred as a result of the use of information contained within this document, including, but not limited to, — errors, omissions, or inaccuracies.

Table of Contents

EASY ROASTED ASPARAGUS 8

BLUEBERRY CREAM CHEESE CROISSANT BAKE 10

GARLIC AND HERB ARTISAN BREAD 12

KETO LOW-CARB ONION RINGS 14

HILTON DOUBLETREE HOTEL CHOCOLATE CHIP COOKIES 17

KOREAN AIR FRIED GREEN BEANS 19

GENERAL TSO TOFU 21

ROASTED BARLEY TEA 23

ROASTED CINNAMON SUGAR ORANGE 24

AIR FRYER SWEET POTATO FRIES 26

BLUEBERRY CREAM CHEESE MUFFINS 28

AIR FRYER BBQ BRUSSELS SPROUTS 30

HOTTEOK KOREAN SWEET PANCAKES 32

PARMESAN SUGAR SNAP PEAS 34

AIR FRYER ROASTED ALMONDS 36

GOCHUJANG LOTUS ROOT 38

KOREAN BBQ LOTUS ROOT 40

HONEY SESAME TOFU 42

RASPBERRY NUTELLA TOAST CUPS 44

TURNIP FRIES 46

HOME FRIES 48

BBQ BABY CORN 50

AIR FRIED BANANA.. 52

SWEET AND SOUR BRUSSEL SPROUTS 54

AIR FRYER ITALIAN ROASTED POTATOES 56

MOZZARELLA STUFFED MUSHROOMS... 58

RED BEAN WHEEL PIE (IMAGAWAYAKI)... 60

CRISPY CURRY CHICKPEAS 62

CHEESY CAULIFLOWER CROQUETTES 64

CURRY ROASTED CAULIFLOWER 66

VIETNAMESE VEGETARIAN EGG MEATLOAF 68

BROCCOLI AND MUSHROOM OMELETTE 71

TARO BALLS WITH SALTED EGG YOLKS 73

BLACK PEPPER MUSHROOM 75

VEGETARIAN GRILLED UNAGI 77

AIR FRIED BUTTON MUSHROOMS 79

MARINATED KOREAN BBQ TOFU 81

BUTTERED GREEN BEANS 83

MATCHA RED BEAN TOAST 84

CUMIN SPICED TOFU SKEWERS 86

MAPLE BANANA FRENCH TOAST BAKE 88

WASABI AVOCADO FRIES 90

ROASTED GARLIC... 93

TOFU WITH BAMBOO SHOOTS 94

OYSTER SAUCE MUSHROOM 96

FRIED OKRA WITH SRIRACHA MAYO 98

MISO TOFU 100

MAPLE WALNUT BISCOTTI 102

KIMCHI TOFU STIR FRY 104

CHEESY ROASTED POTATOES 106

Easy Roasted Asparagus

Prep Time: 5 mins

Cook Time: 8 mins

Ingredients

- 1 pound asparagus ends trimmed (about 500g)
- 1/4 tsp sea salt or to taste
- 1/8 teaspoon black pepper or to taste
- 1 tablespoon extra virgin olive oil

Instructions

Rinse the asparagus and drain.

Put the asparagus on a large plate and drizzle olive oil on it and season with salt, pepper. Mix gently. Line the fryer basket with a grill mat or a sheet of lightly greased aluminum foil.

Put the asparagus in the fryer basket, without stacking if possible, and air fry at 360F (180C) for about 6-8 minutes until tender.

Nutrition

Calories: 54kcal | Carbohydrates: 4g | Protein: 3g | Fat: 4g | Saturated Fat: 1g | Sodium: 148mg | Potassium: 229mg | Fiber: 2g | Sugar: 2g |Vitamin C: 6mg | Calcium: 27mg | Iron: 2mg

Blueberry Cream Cheese Croissant Bake

Prep Time: 10 mins

Cook Time: 20 mins

Ingredients

- 1/2 tube crescent dough (4 crescents) (or puff pastry sheets)
- 1/2 cup blueberry
- 4 oz cream cheese (約 113g)
- 1/3 cup sugar
- 1 egg
- 1/2 teaspoon vanilla
- 2 tablespoon milk

Instructions

Roll the crescent dough into the shape of a crescent and set it aside. Lightly grease a shallow baking dish and set it aside.

In an electric mixer, cream together cream cheese and sugar until fluffy.

Add in milk, egg, and vanilla and mix until well combined and pour the mixture into the baking dish. Place the crescents on top and sprinkle the blueberries into the dish.

Air fry at 280F (140C) for 18-20 minutes until the egg is set and the crescent rolls are golden brown.

Nutrition

Calories: 206kcal | Carbohydrates: 22g | Protein: 4g | Fat: 12g | Saturated Fat: 6g | Cholesterol: 73mg | Sodium: 138mg | Potassium: 78mg | Fiber: 1g | Sugar: 20g | Vitamin C: 2mg | Calcium: 42mg | Iron: 1mg

Garlic And Herb Artisan Bread

Prep Time: 2 hrs

Cook Time: 20 mins

Ingredients

- 1 cup water about 95F (35C)
- 1/2 tablespoon instant dry yeast
- 1/2 tablespoon salt
- 2 1/4 cup all-purpose flour
- 2 teaspoon garlic powder or to taste
- 1/2 teaspoon onion powder
- 1 teaspoon thyme
- 1/2 teaspoon dried parsley

Instructions

In a medium bowl, gently stir the water and yeast.

In a large mixing bowl, combine all dry ingredients and mix well.

Pour the yeast and water mixture into the mixing bowl containing the dry ingredients and mix well. Cover the mixing bowl with a damp towel and let rise for about 2 hours or until the dough rose and double in size.

Line a 7-inch cake barrel with parchment paper. Sprinkle a little flour onto the parchment paper.

Use a spatula to punch down the dough then transfer the dough to the cake barrel. Sprinkle some flour on top and let it rise for about 30 minutes.

If the air fryer you use has a detachable basket, pour about 3 tablespoons of water into the bottom of the outer basket. Preheat the air fryer at 400F (200C) for about 4 minutes.

Put the cake barrel inside the fryer basket and air fryer at 400F (200C) for about 10-12 minutes until the bread has a nice golden-brown crust.

Turn the bread over and air fry again at 400F (200C) for another 4-6 minutes until the crust is golden brown. Try knocking on the bread, if it sounds hollow then it is cooked through on the inside.

Let cool on a wired rack for about 10-15 minutes before slicing.

Nutrition

Calories: 176kcal | Carbohydrates: 37g | Protein: 5g | Fat: 1g | Saturated Fat: 1g | Sodium: 585mg | Potassium: 62mg

| Fiber: 1g | Sugar: 1g | Vitamin C: 1mg | Calcium: 7mg | Iron: 2mg

Keto Low-Carb Onion Rings

Prep Time 15 mins

Cook Time 10 mins

Total Time 25 mins

Ingredients

- large vidalia onion peeled Mine weighed 12oz. See notes for other onions to substitute.
- 1/2 cup King Arthur Keto Wheat Flour Blend See notes for substitutions.
- 1 teaspoon garlic powder
- 1 teaspoon smoked paprika
- salt and pepper to taste
- The breading will be very bland without salt. Be sure to season.
- 1 egg Beaten
- 1 1/2 cup crushed pork rinds

Instructions

Cut the stems off both sides of the onion. Cut the onion into 1/2 inch thick rounds. Onions are very wobbly. Be careful while slicing and use a mandolin if necessary. Try to stabilize the onion before you slice.

Set up a cooking station using 3 bowls large enough to dredge the onions. Add the Keto Wheat Flour Blend to a bowl. Season the flour with the smoked paprika, garlic powder, salt, and pepper to taste.

Add the beaten egg to a bowl.

Add the crushed pork rinds to a bowl.

Dredge the sliced onions in the flour, then the egg, and then the crushed pork rinds. Keep a moist kitchen towel handy for you hands. They will get sticky. It may look like you aren't getting much flour onto the rings. Ensure the full ring is submerged in flour and coated, you may need to do a couple of passes in the flour.

Air Fryer Instructions

Spray the air fryer basket with cooking oil.

Place the breaded onion rings in the air fryer. Do not stack them. Cook in batches if needed. (Optional to spray the onion rings with cooking oil here.)

Cook for 8-10 minutes on 400 degrees. I found that my onion rings did not need a flip. Check in on yours to determine both sides are golden brown and crisp. Flip if necessary.

Baking Instructions

Preheat oven to 400 degrees.

Line a sheet pan with parchment paper. Place the breaded onion rings on the parchment paper. Bake for 10 minutes. Flip the onion rings. (Optional to spray the onion rings with cooking oil here.) Bake for an additional 10-12 minutes or until crisp.

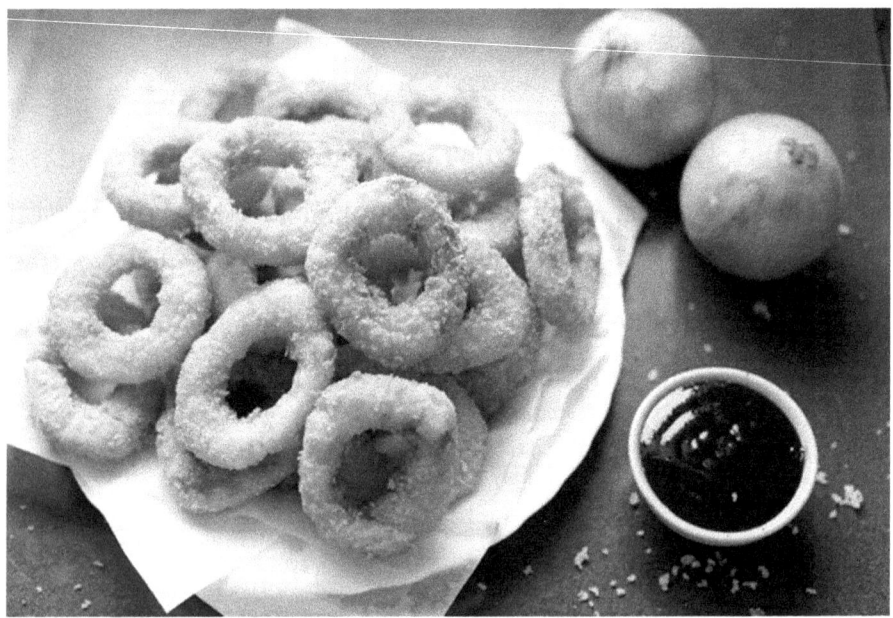

Hilton DoubleTree Hotel Chocolate Chip Cookies

Prep Time: 10 mins

Cook Time: 1 hr

Ingredients

- 1/2 cup butter softened
- 1/3 cup granulated sugar
- 1/4 cup packed brown sugar
- 1 egg
- 1/2 teaspoons vanilla extract
- 1/8 teaspoon lemon juice
- 1 cup and 2 tablespoons all-purpose flour
- 1/4 cup rolled oats
- 1/2 teaspoon baking soda
- 1/2 teaspoon salt
- Pinch cinnamon
- 1 1/4 cup semi-sweet chocolate chips
- 1 cup chopped walnuts

Instructions

Cream butter, sugar, and brown sugar in the bowl of a stand mixer on medium speed for about 2 minutes.

Add eggs, vanilla, and lemon juice, blending with mixer on low speed for 30 seconds, then medium speed for about 2 minutes, or until light and fluffy, scraping down bowl.

With the mixer on low speed, add flour, oats, baking soda, salt, and cinnamon, blending for about 45 seconds. Don't overmix.

Remove bowl from mixer and stir in chocolate chips and walnuts. Line the fryer basket with a grill mat or a sheet of parchment paper.

Scoop about one tablespoon of dough onto a baking sheet lined with parchment paper about 2 inches apart.

Air fry at 260F (130C) for 18-20 minutes.

Remove from the air fryer and cool on a wired rack for about 1/2 hour.

Nutrition

Calories: 397kcal | Carbohydrates: 30g | Protein: 5g | Fat: 29g | Saturated Fat: 15g | Cholesterol: 55mg | Sodium: 154mg | Potassium: 182mg | Fiber: 3g | Sugar: 17g | Vitamin C: 1mg | Calcium: 34mg | Iron: 2mg

Korean Air Fried Green Beans

Prep Time: 5 mins

Cook Time: 15 mins

Ingredients

- 1 pound green beans (about 500g) washed and dried in a colander
- 1/3 cup Korean BBQ sauce
- 1/2 teaspoon black pepper or to taste
- 2 teaspoon toasted sesame seeds

Instructions

Line the fryer basket with a grill mat or a sheet of lightly greased aluminum foil. In a mixing bowl, mix and coat the green beans with the seasoning ingredients. Transfer all contents in the mixing bowl into the fryer basket.

Air fry at 400F (200C) for 14-16 minutes, stirring a few times in between until the surface is slightly caramelized. When you see the BBQ sauce starts drying up, keep an eye on it, as you don't want the beans to get charred. Therefore, check more frequently towards the end.

Sprinkle some sesame seeds to serve.

Nutrition

Calories: 74kcal | Carbohydrates: 15g | Protein: 3g | Fat: 1g | Saturated Fat: 1g | Sodium: 379mg | Potassium: 250mg | Fiber: 3g | Sugar: 9g | Vitamin C: 14mg | Calcium: 52mg | Iron: 1mg

General Tso Tofu

Prep Time: 2 hrs

Cook Time: 15 mins

Ingredients

- 10 oz firm tofu (about 285g)
- 2 tablespoon thinly sliced green onion
- 1 teaspoon sesame seeds
- Ingredients for the sauce:
- 1 Tablespoon chili oil
- 2 Tablespoon minced garlic
- 1 Tablespoon grated ginger
- 2 Tablespoon soy sauce
- 1 Tablespoon vinegar
- 1 1/2 Tablespoon sugar
- 2 teaspoon corn starch mix with 4 teaspoon water

Instructions

Place a kitchen towel on the counter and place the tofu on top. Put a heavy item, such as a small pot, on top of the tofu for one hour to squeeze out excess water.

Line the fryer basket with a grill mat or a sheet of lightly greased aluminum foil.

Cut tofu into bite-size pieces and put them in a fryer basket without stacking. Spritz them with some oil and air fry at 400F (200C) for about 10-12 minutes, flip them once in the middle.

In the meantime, prepare the sauce by mixing chili oil, minced garlic, grated ginger, soy sauce, vinegar, and sugar.

Heat the sauce in a wok and bring it to a boil. Mix corn starch with water and add it to the sauce in the wok. Stir constantly until the sauce thickens.

When the tofu is done, toss them in the wok to coat. Sprinkle some sesame seeds and green onion to serve.

Nutrition

Calories: 129kcal | Carbohydrates: 10g | Protein: 8g | Fat: 7g | Saturated Fat: 1g | Sodium: 507mg | Potassium: 35mg | Fiber: 1g | Sugar: 5g | Vitamin C: 2mg | Calcium: 101mg | Iron: 1mg

Roasted Barley Tea

Prep Time: 5 mins

Cook Time: 35 mins

Ingredients

- 1/2 cup round or pressed barley

Instructions

Rinse the barley, drain and let dry a bit in a colander.

Put barley in a cake barrel and air fry at 400F (175C) for 30-35 minutes, stirring 3-4 times in the middle, until the color turns dark brown.

Let cool completely before use.

In a teapot put one tablespoon of roasted barley with one cup of boiling water. Let sit for at least 10 minutes for it to become fragrant and flavorful

Nutrition

Calories: 41kcal | Carbohydrates: 8g | Protein: 1g | Fat: 1g | Saturated Fat: 1g | Sodium: 1mg | Potassium: 52mg | Fiber: 2g | Sugar: 1g | Calcium: 4mg | Iron: 1mg

Roasted Cinnamon Sugar Orange

Prep Time: 5 mins

Cook Time: 5 mins

Ingredients

- 4 Oranges
- 1/2 tsp cinnamon
- 2 tsp brown sugar

Instructions

Mix cinnamon and sugar and set aside.

Cut each half of the orange in half. Then, take a serrated knife to cut along the inner edges of the orange rind.

Sprinkle the cinnamon sugar the orange.

Air fry at 400F (200C) for about 4-5 minutes. Serve warm by itself or over ice cream.

Nutrition

Calories: 70kcal | Carbohydrates: 18g | Protein: 1g | Fat: 1g | Saturated Fat: 1g | Sodium: 1mg | Potassium: 237mg | Fiber: 3g | Sugar: 14g | Vitamin A: 295IU | Vitamin C: 70mg | Calcium: 52mg | Iron: 1mg

Air Fryer Sweet Potato Fries

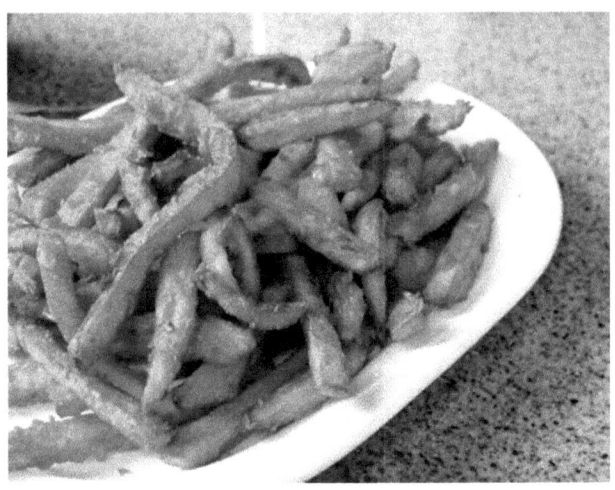

Prep Time: 5 mins

Cook Time: 15 mins

Ingredients

- 1 pound sweet potatoes peeled (about 500g)
- 1 tablespoon olive oil
- 1/2 teaspoon garlic powder
- 1/2 teaspoon onion powder
- 1/2 teaspoon paprika
- 1/2 teaspoon salt or to taste
- 1/4 teaspoon white pepper powder
- 1/2 teaspoon dried basil flakes to garnish

Instructions

Line the fryer basket with a grill mat or a sheet of lightly greased aluminum foil. Cut the sweet potato into 1/4 inch sticks.

In a large mixing bowl, toss the sweet potato sticks with all other ingredients, except dried basil flakes. Place the sweet potato sticks inside the fryer basket without stacking, if possible. Air fry at 380F (190C) for 14-16 minutes, stirring once in the middle until the edges look nice and crisp.

Sprinkle some dried basil to serve.

Nutrition

Calories: 132kcal | Carbohydrates: 24g | Protein: 2g | Fat: 4g | Saturated Fat: 1g | Sodium: 354mg | Potassium: 382mg | Fiber: 3g | Sugar: 5g |Vitamin C: 3mg | Calcium: 34mg | Iron: 1mg

Blueberry Cream Cheese Muffins

Prep Time: 10 mins

Cook Time: 10 mins

Ingredients

- 1 1/2 cups all-purpose flour
- 1/2 cup white sugar
- 1/2 teaspoon salt
- 2 teaspoons baking powder
- 1/4 cup vegetable oil
- 8 oz cream cheese (about 225g) softened at room temperature
- 1 egg
- 1/2 teaspoon vanilla extract
- 1/3 cup milk
- 1 cup fresh blueberries

Instructions

Grease muffin cups or line with muffin liners.

In a large bowl, combine flour, sugar, salt, and baking powder.

In a large mixing bowl, cream together vegetable oil, cream cheese, egg, and vanilla extract. Then, add in milk and all the dried ingredients and mix until well combined.

Fold in blueberries. Scoop the mixture into the muffin tins, about 3/4 full.

Air fry at 320F (160C) for about 12-14 minutes until done, and the toothpick comes out clean.

Nutrition

Calories: 421kcal | Carbohydrates: 47g | Protein: 7g | Fat: 24g | Saturated Fat: 15g | Cholesterol: 70mg | Sodium: 334mg | Potassium: 267mg | Fiber: 1g | Sugar: 21g | Vitamin C: 2mg | Calcium: 119mg | Iron: 2mg

Air Fryer BBQ Brussels Sprouts

Prep Time: 5 mins

Cook Time: 25 mins

Ingredients

- 1 pound Brussels sprouts about 500g
- 2 tsp olive oil
- 1/8 tsp black pepper or to taste
- 1/4 cup BBQ sauce American-style BBQ sauce (such as the Sweet Baby Ray's BBQ sauce)
- 1/4 cup Parmesan cheese or to taste

Instructions

Rinse the Brussels sprouts with cold water and let dry in a colander. Trim off the ends and cut them in half.

In a large mixing bowl, toss the Brussels sprouts, olive oil, and black pepper. Then, wrap them in aluminum foil and air fry at 380F (190C) for about about 16 minutes.

Mix in the BBQ sauce and air fry again at 360F (180C) for 5-6 minutes, stirring once in the middle until the surface is slightly caramelized.

Sprinkle some Parmesan cheese to serve.

Nutrition

Calories: 122kcal | Carbohydrates: 18g | Protein: 6g | Fat: 4g | Saturated Fat: 1g | Cholesterol: 4mg | Sodium: 312mg | Potassium: 483mg | Fiber: 4g | Sugar: 8g | Vitamin C: 96mg | Calcium: 128mg | Iron: 2mg

Hotteok Korean Sweet Pancakes

Prep Time: 2 hrs 30 mins

Cook Time: 10 mins

Ingredients

Ingredients For The Dough:

- 1 1/4 cup all-purpose flour
- 1/2 tsp salt
- 1 tsp white sugar
- 1 tsp instant dry yeast
- 1/2 cup lukewarm milk

Ingredients for the filling:

- 1/4 cup brown sugar
- 1/4 tsp cinnamon powder
- 1/4 cup chopped walnuts

Instructions

In a mixing bowl, mix all the dough ingredients with a spatula.

Lightly cover the bowl with saran wrap and let the dough rise for about 1-2 hours or until the dough doubles in size.

Punch the dough down several times to release the air in the dough. Then, cover with saran wrap again and let it rest for about 20 minutes.

In the meantime, mix all the filling ingredients in a bowl and set aside.

Line the fryer basket with a grill mat or a sheet of lightly greased aluminum foil.

Rub some cooking oil in your hands and take the dough out from the bowl. Roll the dough into a cylinder shape on the counter surface then cut it into six equal pieces. Roll each piece into a ball.

Take one ball of dough and flatten it between the palms of your hand. Scoop about 1 tablespoon of filling and wrap it inside the dough. Place the dough inside the fryer basket, leaving about 2 inches between the balls. Repeat until done.

Press the balls down with the palm of your hand. Spritz some oil on top and air fry at 300F (150C) for 8-10 minutes, flip once in the middle until the surface is golden brown.

Nutrition

Calories: 137kcal | Carbohydrates: 24g | Protein: 4g | Fat: 3g | Saturated Fat: 1g | Cholesterol: 2mg | Sodium: 155mg |

Potassium: 81mg | Fiber: 1g | Sugar: 8g | Calcium: 29mg | Iron: 1mg

Parmesan Sugar Snap Peas

Prep Time: 5 mins

Cook Time: 10 mins

Ingredients

- 1/2 pound sugar snap peas (about 250g)
- 1 tsp olive oil
- 1/4 cup panko breadcrumbs (optional)
- 1/4 cup parmesan cheese
- Salt and pepper to taste
- 2 tbsp minced garlic

Instructions

Remove and discard the stem end and string from each pea pod. Then, rinse and drained in a colander. Line the fryer basket with a grill mat or a sheet of lightly greased aluminum foil.

In a large mixing bowl, toss the snap peans with olive oil, panko breadcrumbs, half of the parmesan cheese, and salt and pepper.

Put the snap pea mixture into the fryer basket and air fry at 360F for about 4 minutes. Stir in the minced garlic then air fry again at 360F (180C) for another 4-5 minutes.

Sprinkle the rest of the parmesan cheese to serve.

Nutrition

Calories: 78kcal | Carbohydrates: 9g | Protein: 5g | Fat: 3g | Saturated Fat: 1g | Cholesterol: 4mg | Sodium: 131mg | Potassium: 129mg | Fiber: 2g | Sugar: 3g | Vitamin C: 35mg | Calcium: 112mg | Iron: 1mg

Air Fryer Roasted Almonds

Prep Time: 1 min

Cook Time: 15 mins

Ingredients

- 1 cup raw almonds

Instructions

Put raw almonds in bakeware, air fry at 320F (160C) for 10-12 minutes, stirring twice in the middle to ensure they roast evenly.

Let cool completely before serving.

Nutrition

Calories: 206kcal | Carbohydrates: 8g | Protein: 8g | Fat: 18g | Saturated Fat: 1g | Sodium: 1mg | Potassium: 252mg | Fiber: 4g | Sugar: 1g | Calcium: 94mg | Iron: 1mg

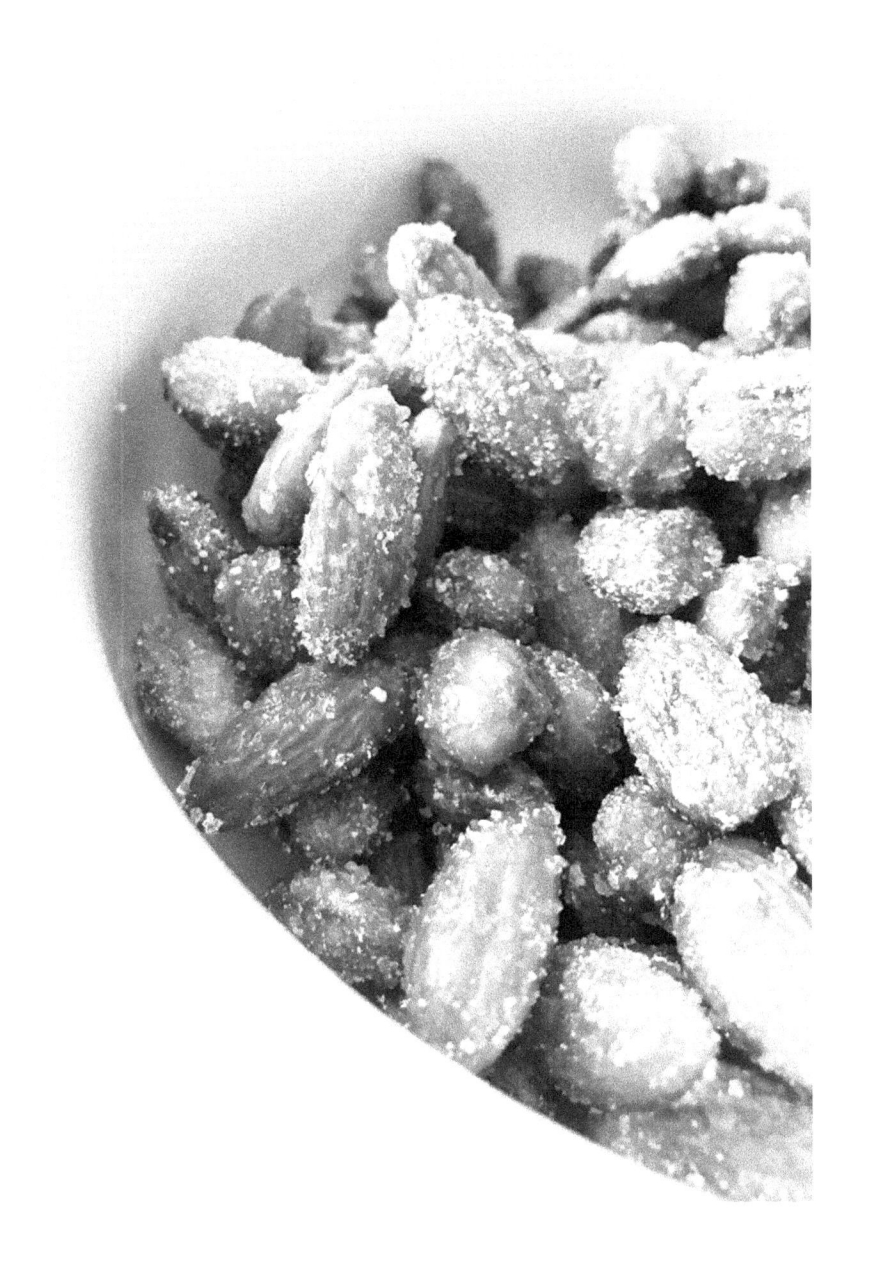

Gochujang Lotus Root

Prep Time: 10 mins

Cook Time: 10 mins

Ingredients

- 1/2 pound lotus root sliced
- about 1/4 inch thick (about 250g)
- 1 tablespoon Gochujang Korean hot pepper paste
- 1 tablespoon soy sauce
- 4 tablespoon honey
- 2 teaspoon apple cider vinegar
- 1 teaspoon sesame seed

Instructions

In a Ziploc bag, mix Gochujang, soy sauce, honey, and apple cider vinegar. Add lotus roots to the bag and mix. Seal the bag and marinate for at least one hour or best overnight.

Line the fryer basket with a grill mat or a sheet of lightly greased aluminum foil.

Put the lotus root slices in the fryer basket without stacking. Air fry at 380F (190C) for about 10 minutes, flip once in the middle until the surface looks slightly caramelized.

In the meantime, transfer the marinade from the bag to a wok or saucepan and bring it to a boil. Stir constantly until the sauce thickens.

Toss the lotus root with the sauce. Then, sprinkle some sesame seeds and scallion to serve.

Nutrition

Calories: 116kcal | Carbohydrates: 29g | Protein: 2g | Fat: 1g | Saturated Fat: 1g | Sodium: 276mg | Potassium: 351mg | Fiber: 3g | Sugar: 18g | Vitamin C: 26mg | Calcium: 30mg | Iron: 1mg

Korean BBQ Lotus Root

Prep Time: 5 mins

Cook Time: 10 mins

Ingredients

- 1/3 cup Korean BBQ Sauce
- 1/2 pound Lotus root cut into 1/4 inch slices (about 250g)
- 1 teaspoon sesame seeds
- 2 tablespoon scallion

Instructions

Marinate lotus in Korean BBQ sauce for at least 1 hour or best overnight.

Line the fryer basket with a grill mat or a sheet of lightly greased aluminum foil.

Put the lotus root slices in the fryer basket without stacking. Air fry at 380F (190C) for about 6-8 minutes, flip once in the middle until the surface looks slightly caramelized.

In the meantime, transfer the marinade from the bag to a wok or saucepan and bring it to a boil. Stir constantly until the sauce thickens.

Toss the lotus root with the sauce. Then, sprinkle some sesame seeds and scallion to serve.

Nutrition

Calories: 79kcal | Carbohydrates: 17g | Protein: 3g | Fat: 1g | Saturated Fat: 1g | Sodium: 396mg | Potassium: 326mg | Fiber: 3g | Sugar: 6g | Vitamin A: 30IU | Vitamin C: 26mg | Calcium: 30mg | Iron: 1mg

Honey Sesame Tofu

Prep Time: 1 hr

Cook Time: 30 mins

Ingredients

- 1 box firm tofu about
- 1 pound or 500g
- 1/3 cup honey
- 1/3 cup soy sauce
- 1/4 cup ketchup
- 1/4 cup brown sugar
- 1/4 cup rice vinegar
- 1 tsp sesame oil
- 2 Tbsp minced garlic
- 1 Tbsp sesame seeds for garnish or to taste
- 1/4 cup scallions for garnish or to taste

Instructions

Wrap the tofu in a cheesecloth. Place a heavy pan on top for about 30 minutes. Then, place the tofu in the freezer for at least 6 hours.

Remove the tofu from the freezer and use the defrost function of the microwave for about 10 minutes. After that, repeat step one to squeeze out excess water.

In the meantime, take a large bowl to mix and combine honey, soy sauce, ketchup, brown sugar, vinegar, sesame oil, and garlic. Scoop about 1/2 cup of the marinade and set aside.

Use hands to break the tofu into bite-size pieces and put them inside the large bowl containing the marinade. Stir and let the tofu marinate for at least 30 minutes.

Line the fryer basket with a grill mat or sheet of lightly greased aluminum foil.

Put the tofu pieces inside the fryer basket without stacking and air fry at 400F (200C) for 14-16 minutes, stir once in the middle until the edges of tofu looks a bit caramelized.

While air frying, use a wok or a frying pan to bring the sauce to a boil. Stir constantly until the sauce thickens.

When the tofu is done, toss in the wok to coat. Sprinkle some sesame seeds and scallions to serve.

Nutrition

Calories: 281kcal | Carbohydrates: 46g | Protein: 12g | Fat: 6g | Saturated Fat: 1g | Sodium: 1227mg | Potassium: 164mg | Fiber: 1g | Sugar: 41g | Vitamin C: 3mg | Calcium: 170mg | Iron: 2mg

Raspberry Nutella Toast Cups

Prep Time: 5 mins

Cook Time: 10 mins

Ingredients

- 6 pieces of bread
- 2 tbsp unsalted butter melted
- 1/4 cup Nutella or to taste
- 1/2 cup Raspberry or to taste
- 2 tbsp powdered sugar optional

Instructions

Trim off the sides of the toast and save for them for other uses such as croutons or bread pudding. Flatten the toast with a rolling pin and brush a thin layer of butter to both sides.

Place each of the toast inside a muffin tin and press down against the walls of the tin. Air fry at 320F (160C) for about 7-8 minutes until the toast becomes golden brown.

Spoon some Nutella into the bread cup and spread it inside of the cup. Finally, place the raspberries inside the cup. Dust the cups with powdered sugar if desired.

Nutrition

Calories:196kcal | Carbohydrates: 24g | Protein: 2g | Fat: 10g | Saturated Fat: 9g | Cholesterol: 7mg | Sodium: 21mg | Potassium: 132mg | Fiber: 3g | Sugar: 20g | Vitamin C: 5mg | Calcium: 32mg | Iron: 1mg

Turnip Fries

Prep Time: 30 mins

Cook Time: 15 mins

Ingredients

- 1/2 pound turnip peeled and cut into sticks
- 1/4 tsp salt
- 2 teaspoon olive oil
- 1/4 tsp paprika
- 1/4 tsp onion powder
- 1/8 tsp white pepper powder or to taste
- 1/8 tsp cayenne pepper or to taste (optional)

Instructions

In a mixing bowl, toss the turnip sticks with salt. Let it rest for about 20 minutes to draw some of the water out. Discard the excess water in the bowl.

Toss the turnips sticks in olive oil to coat. Then, add in the rest of the ingredients and toss. Put the turnip sticks into the fryer basket and try to spread them out as much as possible.

Air fry at 380F (190C) for 10-12 minutes, shake basket a couple of times in between until the surface looks crisp and golden brown.

Serve immediately. Sprinkle some dried basil if desired.

Nutrition

Calories: 69kcal | Carbohydrates: 8g | Protein: 1g | Fat: 4g | Saturated Fat: 1g | Sodium: 367mg | Potassium: 217mg | Fiber: 2g | Sugar: 4g | Vitamin A: 175IU | Vitamin C: 24mg | Calcium: 34mg | Iron: 1mg

Home Fries

Prep Time: 5 mins

Cook Time: 10 mins

Ingredients

- 1 russet potato
- 1 tbsp olive oil
- 1/2 tsp salt or to taste
- 1/2 tsp paprika
- 1/4 tsp black pepper
- 1/4 tsp cayenne pepper (optional)

Instructions

Peel and dice the potato into 1/2 inch pieces. Soak the potato in cold water for about 10-15 minutes. Drain.

Toss the potato in olive oil. Then, add the remaining ingredients and toss.

Line the fryer basket with a grill mat or a sheet of lightly greased aluminum foil.

Spread the diced potato inside the fryer basket. Air fry at 380F (190C) for about 10-12 minutes, stir twice in the middle until the surface is crispy and golden brown.

Nutrition

Calories: 84kcal | Carbohydrates: 9g | Protein: 2g | Fat: 5g | Saturated Fat: 1g | Sodium: 395mg | Potassium: 293mg | Fiber: 2g | Sugar: 1g | Vitamin C: 8mg | Calcium: 21mg | Iron: 2mg

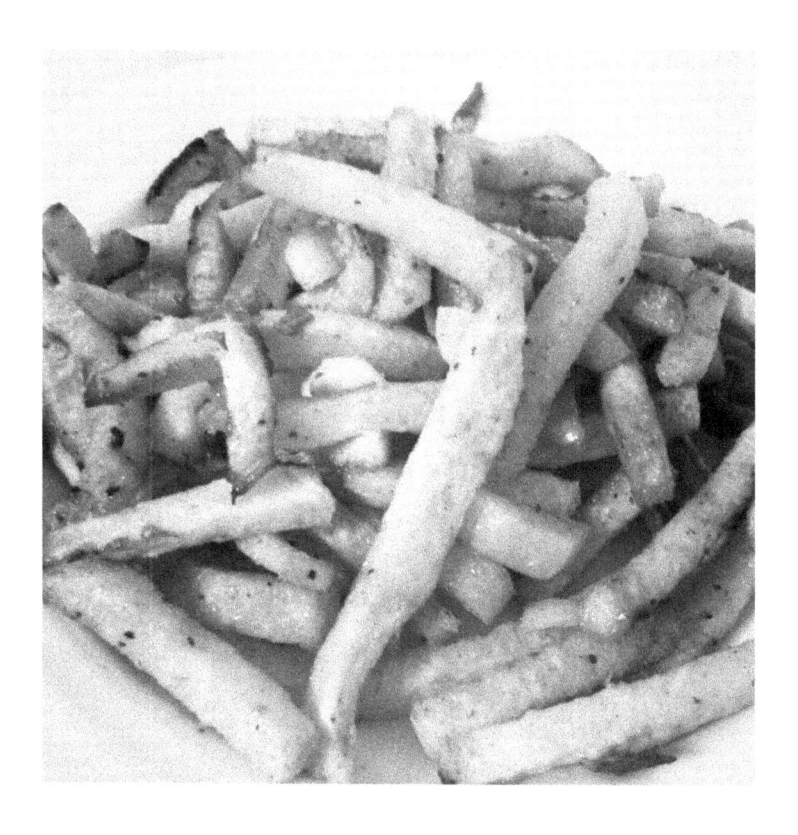

BBQ Baby Corn

Prep Time: 5 mins

Cook Time: 10 mins

Ingredients

- 1 can baby corn drained and rinse with cold water
- 1/4 cup Korean BBQ sauce or to taste **
- 1/2 tsp Sriracha or to taste optional

Instructions

Line the fryer basket with a grill mat or a sheet of lightly greased aluminum foil.

In a large bowl, mix the Korean BBQ sauce and Sriracha. Roll the baby corn in the sauce and place them inside the fryer basket without stacking.

Air fry at 400F (200C) for about 8-10 minutes, brush some more sauce onto baby corn if necessary until the sauce on the surface is slightly caramelized.

Nutrition

Serving: 0.5cup | Calories: 98kcal | Carbohydrates: 18g | Protein: 2g | Fat: 1g | Sodium: 325mg | Sugar: 8g | Vitamin C: 1mg

Air Fried Banana

Prep Time: 5 mins

Cook Time: 10 mins

Ingredients

- 1 ripe banana cut into 1/2 inch slices
- 1/4 tsp cinnamon
- 1/2 tsp brown sugar
- 1 tbsp Granola to taste
- 1 tbsp Chopped toasted nuts to taste

Instructions

In a small bowl, mix the cinnamon and brown sugar and set aside.

Lightly grease a shallow baking pan. Place the banana slices into the pan. Spray some oil onto the banana and sprinkle some cinnamon sugar. Air fry at 400F (200C) for about 4-5 minutes.

Sprinkle some granola and nuts over the banana to serve.

Nutrition

Calories: 113kcal | Carbohydrates: 19g | Protein: 2g | Fat: 4g | Saturated Fat: 1g | Sodium: 3mg | Potassium: 253mg | Fiber: 2g | Sugar: 9g | Vitamin A: 38IU | Vitamin C: 5mg | Iron: 1mg

Sweet And Sour Brussel Sprouts

Prep Time: 5 mins

Cook Time: 20 mins

Ingredients

- 1 pound Brussels sprouts (about 500g)
- 1 tsp olive oil
- 1 tbsp minced garlic
- 1/4 tsp salt or to taste
- 2 tbsp Thai Sweet Chili Sauce
- 2-3 tsp lime juice

Instructions

Rinse the Brussels sprouts with cold water and let dry in a colander. Trim off the ends and cut them in half.

In a large mixing bowl, toss the Brussels sprouts and garlic with olive oil and wrap them in aluminum foil. Air fry at 380F (190C) for about about 18 minutes.

In a mixing bowl, toss the Sprouts with Thai Sweet Chili Sauce and lime juice to serve.

Nutrition

Calories: 79kcal | Carbohydrates: 15g | Protein: 4g | Fat: 1g | Saturated Fat: 1g | Sodium: 259mg | Potassium: 441mg | Fiber: 4g | Sugar: 7g | Vitamin A: 855IU | Vitamin C: 98mg | Calcium: 51mg | Iron: 2mg

Air Fryer Italian Roasted Potatoes

Prep Time: 8 mins

Cook Time: 10 mins

Total Time: 15 mins

Ingredient

- ½ Pound mini potatoes
- 2 teaspoons extra-virgin olive oil
- 2 teaspoons dry italian-style salad dressing mix
- Salt and white pepper to taste

Instructions

Preheat the air fryer to 400 degrees F (200 degrees C).

Wash and dry potatoes. Trim edges to make a flat surface on both ends.

Combine extra-virgin olive oil and salad dressing mix in a large bowl. Add potatoes and toss until potatoes are well coated. Place in a single layer into the air fryer basket. Cook in batches if necessary. Air fry until potatoes are golden brown, 5 to 7 minutes. Flip potatoes and air fry for an additional 2 to 3 minutes. Season with salt and pepper.

Nutrition Facts

Calories: 132; Protein 2.3g; Carbohydrates 20.3g; Fat 4.8g; Sodium 166.8mg.

Mozzarella Stuffed Mushrooms

Prep Time: 5 mins

Cook Time: 10 mins

Ingredients

- 8 medium to large button mushrooms wiped clean and stem removed
- 3-4 tbsp Korean BBQ sauce
- 1/3 cup mozzarella cheese
- Olive oil spray
- 1/2 tsp basil flakes

Instructions

Line the fryer basket with a grill mat or a sheet of lightly greased aluminum foil.

Scoop about 1/2 teaspoon of Korean BBQ sauce into the mushroom. Then, stuff the mushroom with the desired amount of mozzarella cheese.

Place the mushrooms inside the fryer basket. Spray the mushrooms with some olive oil and air fry at 380F (190C) for about 4-5 minutes until the cheese is golden brown.

Sprinkle some basil flakes to serve if desired.

Nutrition

Calories: 74kcal | Carbohydrates: 7g | Protein: 5g | Fat: 3g | Saturated Fat: 2g | Cholesterol: 10mg | Sodium: 360mg | Potassium: 170mg | Fiber: 1g | Sugar: 5g| Vitamin C: 1mg | Calcium: 67mg | Iron: 1mg

Red Bean Wheel Pie (Imagawayaki)

Prep Time: 10 mins

Cook Time: 10 mins

Ingredients

- 2 tbsp melted butter
- 2 eggs
- 2 tbsp sugar
- 1 tbsp honey
- 1/4 tsp vanilla extract
- 1/4 cup milk
- 1 cupcake flour
- 3/4 tsp baking powder
- 6 tbsp mashed sweetened red bean canned or homemade filling to taste

Instructions

Lightly grease 4 ramekins with butter and place them in the fryer basket. Preheat at 400F (200C) for 2 minutes.

In a large bowl, use a whisk to mix the egg, sugar, vanilla extract, and honey. Add in milk and whisk until the mixture is homogeneous. Finally, add in the sifted cake flour and baking powder. Continue to mix until everything is well blended.

The total weight of the batter is about 280g. Spoon about 30g into the ramekin. Air fry at 300F (150C) for about 3 minutes.

Take the desired amount of red bean (about 1 1/2 Tablespoon for mine) and roll it into a ball using the palms of your hand. Flatten it into a circular disc that is smaller than the diameter of the ramekin. Place it in the center of the ramekin on top of the pancake. Scoop about 40g of the batter into the ramekins to cover the red beans.

Air fry again at 300F (150C) for about 3 minutes. Brush some butter on top and air fry again at 300F (150C) for 1-2 minutes until the top is slightly golden brown.

Nutrition

Calories: 284kcal | Carbohydrates: 47g | Protein: 8g | Fat: 9g | Saturated Fat: 5g | Cholesterol: 98mg | Sodium: 101mg | Potassium: 157mg | Fiber: 2g | Sugar: 20g | Vitamin A: 318IU | Calcium: 67mg | Iron: 1mg

Crispy Curry Chickpeas

Prep Time: 5 mins

Cook Time: 25 mins

Ingredients

- 2 cups canned chickpeas drained
- 1 teaspoon olive oil
- 1/2 teaspoon curry powder
- 1/4 teaspoon onion powder
- 1/4 teaspoon paprika
- 1/4 teaspoon salt or to taste
- 1/8 teaspoon garlic powder
- 1/8 teaspoon cayenne pepper optional
- 1/8 teaspoon mushroom essence or Hondashi optional

Instructions

Mix all the dry ingredients and set aside.

In a large bowl, toss the chickpeas with olive oil. Then, add in the dry ingredients and toss, making sure all chickpeas are coated with seasoning.

In a lightly greased cake pan or bakeware, air fry the chickpeas at 360F (180C) for about 23-25 minutes, shake the basket 3-4 times in the middle, until the surface is crisp and lightly golden brown.

Pour the chickpeas onto a plate. Let cool completely before serving.

Nutrition

Calories: 166kcal | Carbohydrates: 23g | Protein: 8g | Fat: 5g | Saturated Fat: 1g | Sodium: 747mg | Potassium: 236mg | Fiber: 7g | Sugar: 1g | Vitamin A: 175IU | Calcium: 57mg | Iron: 2mg

Cheesy Cauliflower Croquettes

Prep Time: 15 mins

Cook Time: 10 mins

Ingredients

- 2 cups of cauliflower rice preparation see instruction
- 2 eggs beaten
- 1/2 cup Mexican blend cheese or your favorite cheese
- 1/4 cup grated Parmesan cheese
- 1/4 cup Mozzarella cheese
- 1/3 cup breadcrumbs
- 1 teaspoon garlic powder
- 1 teaspoon dried basil
- 1/2 teaspoon onion powder
- 1/4 teaspoon salt or to taste
- 1/4 teaspoon black pepper or to taste

Instructions

Pulse the cauliflower in the food processor a few times until it is about the size of a grain of rice. Transfer the cauliflower rice to a microwave-safe bowl and microwave for about 5-6 minutes.

In a large bowl, combine the cauliflower rice with all the other ingredients (except sriracha mayonnaise). Shape the mixture into the desired shape.

Line the fryer basket with a grill mat or a sheet of lightly greased aluminum foil.

Place the croquettes in the fryer basket and air fry at 400F (200C) for 8-9 minutes, flip once in the middle, until the surface is golden brown.

Serve with sriracha mayo or your favorite dipping sauce.

Nutrition

Calories: 182kcal | Carbohydrates: 11g | Protein: 12g | Fat: 10g | Saturated Fat: 5g |Sodium: 495mg | Potassium: 218mg | Fiber: 2g | Sugar: 2g | Vitamin C: 24mg | Calcium: 242mg | Iron: 1mg

Curry Roasted Cauliflower

Prep Time: 10 mins

Cook Time: 10 mins

Ingredients

- 1/2 head cauliflower break them into small florets
- 2 teaspoon olive oil
- 1/2 teaspoon curry powder
- 1/4 teaspoon paprika
- 1/4 teaspoon cumin
- 1/4 teaspoon garlic powder
- 1/4 teaspoon sea salt or to taste

Instructions

Put the cauliflower florets in a large microwave-safe bowl and microwave for about 4-5 minutes.

When done, transfer the florets to a large mixing bowl. Add in olive oil and toss. Then, add the rest of the ingredients to the mixing bowl and toss again to coat.

Air fry at 350F (175C) for about 5-6 minutes, shake the basket once in between. until you start seeing browning of the edges.

Nutrition

Calories: 38kcal | Carbohydrates: 4g | Protein: 1g | Fat: 2g | Saturated Fat: 1g | Sodium: 167mg | Potassium: 215mg | Fiber: 2g | Sugar: 1g | Vitamin C: 35mg | Calcium: 16mg | Iron: 1mg

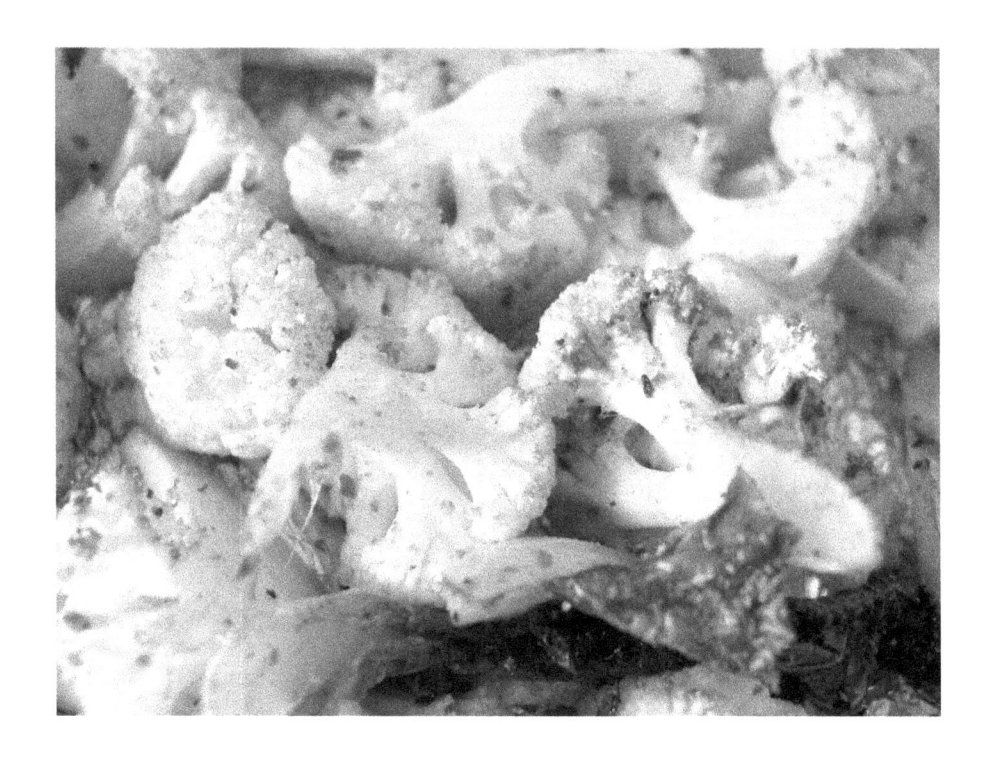

Vietnamese Vegetarian Egg Meatloaf

Prep Time: 30 mins

Cook Time: 20 mins

Ingredients

- 15 g wood ear mushrooms
- 20 g dried shiitake mushrooms
- 4 eggs
- 1/4 cup milk
- small carrot shredded or grated
- 1 tablespoon minced garlic
- 60 g mung bean noodles glass noodles tablespoon fish sauce
- 1/4 teaspoon sugar
- 1/4 teaspoon salt
- 1/4 teaspoon black pepper

Instructions

Soak the shiitake mushrooms and wood ear mushrooms in warm water for about 20 minutes. Once they are softened, squeeze out excess water in the shiitake mushrooms and thinly slice both mushrooms.

Soak mung bean noodles in cold water for about 15 minutes then cut them into 2-inch sections.

Crack 2 whole eggs and 2 egg whites into a large bowl and save the 2 egg yolks in a small bowl for later use.

Add milk into the large bowl and use a whisk to mix until homogenous. Add all the ingredients, except for the egg yolks, into the large bowl and mix.

Spray some oil in a mini loaf pan and pour the egg mixture into the pan. Smooth out the top surface as much as possible since anything that sticks out of the surface will likely be charred during the air frying process.

Air fry at 280F (140C) for 16-18 minutes until the egg is set.

In the meantime, add a pinch of salt into the small bowl containing the egg yolks and mix.

When the egg loaf is done, pour the egg yolk on top and spread it evenly over the egg loaf. Air fry again at 400F (200C) for about 2 minutes until the egg yolks are hardened.

When cool enough to handle, remove the egg loaf from the pan and cut them into 3/4 inch thick slices. Spoon some sauce over it to serve.

Nutrition

Calories: 167kcal | Carbohydrates: 24g | Protein: 8g | Fat: 5g | Saturated Fat: 2g | Cholesterol: 165mg | Sodium: 783mg | Potassium: 300mg | Fiber: 2g | Sugar: 2g | Vitamin C: 2mg | Calcium: 61mg | Iron: 1mg

Broccoli And Mushroom Omelette

Prep Time: 10 mins

Cook Time: 10 mins

Ingredients

- 2 eggs beaten
- 1/4 cup broccoli florets steamed
- 1/4 cup buttoned mushroom sliced
- 1/4 cup shredded cheese Mexican Blend
- 2-3 Tablespoon milk
- 1/8 teaspoon salt and pepper or to taste
- 4-5 slices of pickled jalapeno or to taste (optional)
- Extra cheese to sprinkle

Instructions

Lightly grease a shallow baking pan and set it aside.

In a large bowl, mix the eggs, broccoli, mushroom, 1/4 cup shredded cheese, milk, salt, and pepper, and pour it into the pan. Then, place the jalapeno slices on top (or can be chopped up and mix with the egg mixture).

Air fry at 320F (160C) for about 6-8 minutes. Sprinkle some more cheese on top and air fry again at 320F (160C) for another 2 minutes or so until the eggs are set.

Nutrition

Calories: 121kcal | Carbohydrates: 3g | Protein: 10g | Fat: 8g | Saturated Fat: 4g | Cholesterol: 176mg | Sodium: 323mg | Potassium: 155mg | Fiber: 1g | Sugar: 2g | Vitamin C: 10mg | Calcium: 118mg | Iron: 1mg

Taro Balls With Salted Egg Yolks

Prep Time: 20 mins

Cook Time: 10 mins

Ingredients

- 6 salted egg yolk
- 1 teaspoon rice wine
- 500 g taro steamed
- 50 g corn starch
- 80 g sugar
- 1/4 teaspoon salt
- 2 Tablespoon coconut oil

Instructions

Coat the egg yolk with rice wine and let sit for 10 minutes. Put the egg yolks in shallow bakeware and air fry at 380F (190C) for about 3-4 minutes.

Put all other ingredients in a mixing bowl. Mush and mix all ingredients until the texture is dough-like and without lumps. Alternatively, a food processor can be used as well.

When done, divide this taro dough into 6 equal portions and roll them into round balls. Flatten each ball and put an egg yolk in the middle. Wrap the dough around the egg yolk and roll it into a ball again, making sure there are no cracks or openings.

Line the fryer basket with a grill mat or lightly greased aluminum foil.

Place the taro balls inside the fryer basket. Air fry at 380F (190C) for 8-10 minutes, shake the basket once in the middle until the surface is golden brown.

Nutrition

Calories: 276kcal | Carbohydrates: 44g | Protein: 4g | Fat: 10g | Saturated Fat: 6g | Cholesterol: 195mg | Sodium: 116mg | Potassium: 512mg | Fiber: 3g | Sugar: 14g | Vitamin C: 4mg | Calcium: 59mg | Iron: 1mg

Black Pepper Mushroom

Prep Time: 5 mins

Cook Time: 10 mins

Ingredients

- 8 oz button mushrooms (about 250g) wiped clean, halved, or quartered
- 1 Tablespoon butter melted
- 2 cloves of garlic thinly sliced
- 1 Tablespoon oyster sauce or to taste
- 3/4 teaspoon black pepper or to taste
- 1/4 cup green onion finely sliced

Instructions

Put melted butter and garlic in a cake pan and air fry at 380F (190C) for 2 minutes.

Add the mushroom into the pan and stir. Air fry at 360F (180C) for 3 minutes. Stir in the oyster sauce and black pepper. Air fry again at 360F (180C) for 2-3 minutes.

Sprinkle some green onion to serve.

Nutrition

Calories: 90kcal | Carbohydrates: 7g | Protein: 4g | Fat: 6g | Saturated Fat: 4g | Cholesterol: 15mg | Sodium: 255mg | Potassium: 395mg | Fiber: 2g | Sugar: 3g | Vitamin C: 6mg | Calcium: 14mg | Iron: 1mg

Vegetarian Grilled Unagi

Prep Time: 10 mins

Cook Time: 5 mins

Ingredients

- 1 Chinese eggplant cut in half
- 2 Tablespoon Unagi sauce or Teriyaki sauce or to taste
- 1 teaspoon toasted sesame seeds
- 2 tablespoon thinly sliced green onion

Instructions

Steam the eggplants until tender.

When cool enough to handle, cut the eggplant vertically without cutting through. Then, score the flesh of the eggplants so they look like tiny squares or rectangles.

Line the fryer basket with a grill mat or lightly greased aluminum foil.

Brush both sides of the eggplants with Unagi sauce (or Teriyaki sauce). Place the eggplant into the fryer basket skin side down and air fry at 400F (200C) for about 4-5 minutes.

Sprinkle some sesame seeds and green onion to serve.

Nutrition

Calories: 81kcal | Carbohydrates: 17g | Protein: 4g | Fat: 1g | Saturated Fat: 1g | Sodium: 405mg | Potassium: 565mg | Fiber: 7g | Sugar: 11g | Vitamin C: 6mg | Calcium: 30mg | Iron: 1mg

Air Fried Button Mushrooms

Prep Time: 5 mins

Cook Time: 10 mins

Ingredients

- 10 medium button mushrooms wiped clean with a paper towel and quartered
- 1 egg beaten
- 1/2 cup breadcrumbs
- 1/2 teaspoon garlic powder
- 1/2 teaspoon onion powder
- 1/4 teaspoon dried basil
- 1/4 teaspoon black pepper
- 1/4 teaspoon salt
- Ranch dressing optional

Instructions

Put all the dry ingredients in a large Ziploc bag and shake well.

Dip the mushroom pieces in the egg then drop them into the Ziploc bag. Shake the bag to coat the mushroom pieces with bread crumb mixture.

Shake off excess bread crumbs from the mushroom and place them in the fryer basket. Spray some oil onto the mushrooms and air fry at 400F (200C) for about 3 minutes. Flip the mushrooms and spray some oil again. Air fry at 400F (200C) for another 2-3 minutes.

Serve immediately with ranch dressing or the sauce of your choice.

Nutrition

Calories: 330kcal | Carbohydrates: 48g | Protein: 19g | Fat: 8g | Saturated Fat: 2g | Cholesterol: 164mg | Sodium: 659mg | Potassium: 590mg | Fiber: 4g | Sugar: 8g | Vitamin C: 4mg | Calcium: 123mg | Iron: 5mg

Marinated Korean BBQ Tofu

Prep Time: 2 hrs

Cook Time: 15 mins

Ingredients

- 8 oz firm tofu cut into bite-size cubes
- 1 cup Korean BBQ Sauce
- 2-3 Tablespoon minced garlic
- Thinly sliced scallions and sesame optional

Instructions

In a Ziploc bag or a container with a lid, marinate the tofu with Korean BBQ sauce and grated garlic for at least 2 hours.

Line the fryer basket with a Grill mat or a sheet of lightly greased aluminum foil.

Place the tofu cube inside the fryer basket and air fry at 400F (200C) for 10-12 minutes, flip once in the middle, until the surface is caramelized.

Garnish with scallions and sesame seeds to serve if desired.

Nutrition

Calories: 152kcal | Carbohydrates: 22g | Protein: 9g | Fat: 3g | Saturated Fat: 1g | Sodium: 638mg | Potassium: 49mg | Fiber: 1g | Sugar: 17g | Vitamin C: 1mg | Calcium: 78mg | Iron: 1mg

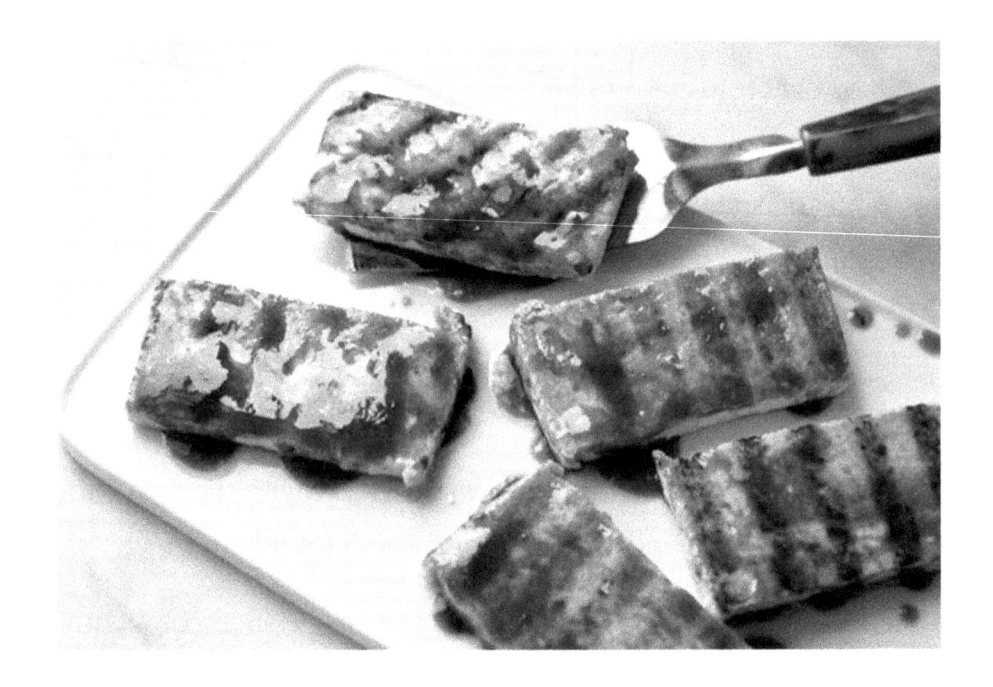

Buttered Green Beans

Prep Time: 5 mins

Cook Time: 10 mins

Ingredients

- 1 pound green beans (about 500g) rinsed and dried
- 1 1/2 Tablespoon unsalted butter melted
- 1/2 teaspoon sea salt
- 1/4 teaspoon black pepper
- 2 Tablespoon chopped garlic

Instructions

Toss the green beans with melted butter, salt, and pepper. Air fry at 350F (175C) for about 4 minutes. Add in the garlic, stir, and air fry again at 350F (175C) for another 3-4 minutes.

Nutrition

Calories: 62kcal | Carbohydrates: 5g | Protein: 2g | Fat: 4g | Saturated Fat: 3g | Cholesterol: 11mg | Sodium: 321mg | Potassium: 211mg | Fiber: 1g | Sugar: 1g |Vitamin C: 28mg | Calcium: 22mg | Iron: 1mg

Matcha Red Bean Toast

Prep Time: 5 mins

Cook Time: 10 mins

Ingredients

- 4 pieces of bread
- 1 Tablespoon unsalted butter softened
- Canned Japanese sweetened red bean (mashed), to taste
- 3 tablespoon matcha green tea powder
- 1 1/4 Tablespoon water

Instructions

In a small bowl, matcha mixes green tea powder with water until it forms a thickened paste. Spread the paste on one piece of bread and the mashed red bean on the other piece (one side only).

Put the two pieces together to make a sandwich.

Spread the softened butter onto the outside of the sandwich on both sides. Stick one toothpick through the sandwich to prevent the displacement of bread during the air frying process.

Air fry at 400F (200C) for about 7-8 minutes, flip once until the surface is golden brown.

Nutrition

Calories: 123kcal | Carbohydrates: 1g | Protein: 12g | Fat: 6g | Saturated Fat: 4g | Cholesterol: 15mg | Sodium: 12mg | Sugar: 1g | Vitamin A: 1300IU | Iron: 4mg

Cumin Spiced Tofu Skewers

Prep Time: 1 hr 10 mins

Cook Time: 15 mins

Ingredients

- 8 oz firm tofu
- 2 Tablespoon soy paste
- 1 Tablespoon olive oil
- 1 Tablespoon cumin
- 1 teaspoon brown sugar
- 1/4 teaspoon cayenne pepper or to taste
- 1/4 Sichuan peppercorn powder or to taste
- 2 tablespoon thinly sliced green onion
- 1 teaspoon toasted sesame seeds

Instructions

Place a kitchen towel on the counter and place the tofu on top. Put a heavy item, such as a small pot, on top of the tofu for one hour to squeeze out excess water.

Soak bamboo skewers in water for at least 10 minutes. Take a metal steamer rack and brush olive oil onto the surface of the rack and put it inside the fryer basket.

In a small bowl, prepare the sauce by mixing all the seasoning ingredients and set aside.

Cut tofu into bite-size pieces and thread them on 2 skewers parallel to each other. Generously brush both sides of the tofu with a layer of the seasoning mixture and place the skewers on top of the steamer rack.

Air fry at 400F (200C) for about 10-12 minutes, brushing more sauce in the middle if necessary, until the surface of the tofu is slightly caramelized.

Sprinkle some sesame seeds and green onion to serve.

Nutrition

Calories: 107kcal | Carbohydrates: 6g | Protein: 6g | Fat: 7g | Saturated Fat: 1g | Sodium: 198mg | Potassium: 27mg | Fiber: 1g | Sugar: 3g | Vitamin A: 101IU | Vitamin C: 1mg | Calcium: 90mg | Iron: 2mg

Maple Banana French Toast Bake

Prep Time: 5 mins

Cook Time: 20 mins

Ingredients

- makes two loaves using 5.75 in x 3 in mini loaf pans
- 2 eggs beaten
- 1/4 cups milk
- 1 Tablespoon brown sugar
- 3 Tablespoon maple syrup
- 1 Tablespoon butter melted
- 1 teaspoon vanilla extract
- 1/4 teaspoon ground cinnamon
- 1 small banana sliced
- 4 slices of bread cubed
- 1/3 cup raw walnut chopped
- Raw chop walnuts to top

Instructions

In a large mixing bowl, mix the eggs, milk, brown sugar, maple syrup, butter, vanilla extract, and cinnamon. When the mixture is well combined, gently stir in bread cubes, banana, and chopped pecans. Scoop the mixture into a lightly greased mini loaf pan and top it with the whole pecan.

Air fry at 280F (140C) for about 12 minutes. Then, carefully remove the loaf from the pan, flip, and place the bread loaf directly on parchment paper (now bottom side up). Air fry at 280F (140C) again for about 6 minutes more.

Nutrition

Calories: 287kcal | Carbohydrates: 36g | Protein: 8g | Fat: 13g | Saturated Fat: 4g | Cholesterol: 91mg | Sodium: 211mg | Potassium: 284mg | Fiber: 3g | Sugar: 18g| Vitamin C: 3mg | Calcium: 94mg | Iron: 2mg

Wasabi Avocado Fries

Prep Time: 5 mins

Cook Time: 10 mins

Ingredients

- 1 avocado pitted and diced
- 1 egg
- 1 1/2 Tablespoon wasabi paste or to taste
- 1/2 teaspoon salt
- 1/2 cup breadcrumbs or Japanese panko
- Lime wedges optional

Instructions

Put the breadcrumbs in a Ziploc bag and set them aside.

In a medium bowl, use a whisk to mix the egg, wasabi paste, and salt until homogenous. Put all the avocado chunks in the egg mixture to coat.

Carefully transfer the avocado into the bag. Shake the bag to coat the avocado with breadcrumbs.

Place the avocado pieces into the fryer basket, spray them with some oil, and air fry at 400F (200C) for about 3 minutes.

Squeeze some lime juice to serve.

Nutrition

Calories: 160kcal | Carbohydrates: 16g | Protein: 5g | Fat: 9g | Saturated Fat: 2g | Cholesterol: 41mg | Sodium: 511mg | Potassium: 325mg | Fiber: 5g | Sugar: 1g | Vitamin C: 8mg | Calcium: 47mg | Iron: 1mg

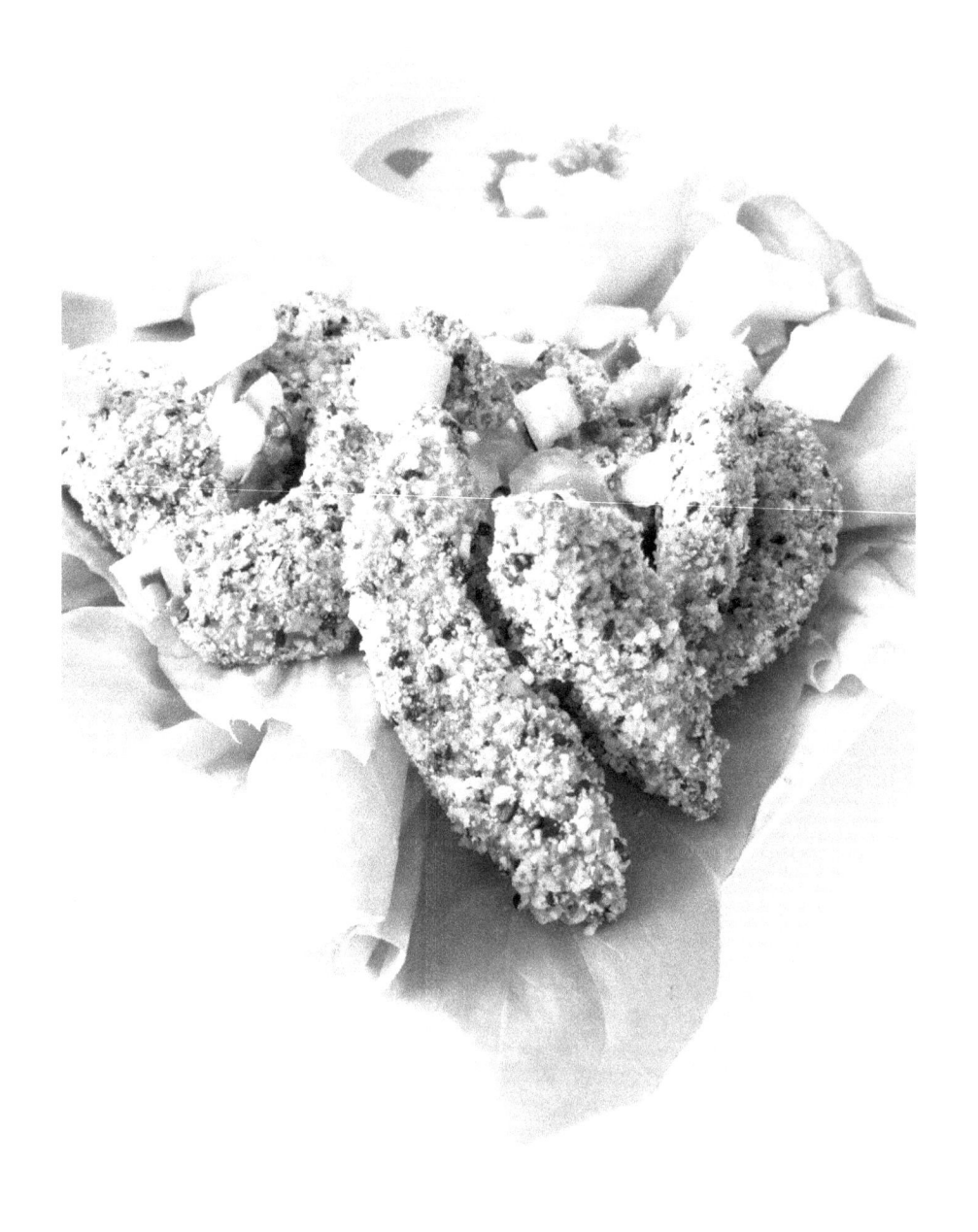

Roasted Garlic

Prep Time: 5 mins

Cook Time: 30 mins

Ingredients

- 3-4 head of garlic
- 2 tbsp Olive oil
- A pinch of salt

Instructions

Slice off the top of garlic. Drizzle some olive oil over it and sprinkle with some salt and pepper. Wrap the garlic with aluminum foil and air fry at 400F (200C) for 25-30 minutes until the garlic is tender and slightly golden brown.

Nutrition

Calories: 65kcal | Carbohydrates: 1g | Protein: 1g | Fat: 7g | Saturated Fat: 1g | Sodium: 1mg | Potassium: 9mg | Sugar: 1g | Vitamin C: 1mg | Calcium: 4mg

Tofu with Bamboo Shoots

Prep Time: 10 mins

Cook Time: 15 mins

Ingredients

Ingredients For Tofu:

- 1 1/4 cup bean curd cut into
- 1/4 inch thick strips
- 1 teaspoon olive oil

Other Ingredients:

- 2 cups bamboo shoots
- 2 Tablespoon garlic minced
- 2 Tablespoon oyster sauce
- 2 Tablespoon soy sauce
- 1 Tablespoon rice wine
- 1 Tablespoon brown sugar
- 1/2 teaspoon Sriracha optional
- 2 green onions cut into one-inch pieces.

Instructions

Line the fryer basket with lightly greased aluminum foil. Toss tofu strips with olive oil then put them into the basket. Air fry at 380F (190C) for about 5 minutes. Add in the bamboo shoots, stir, and air fry again at 380F (190C) for another 3 minutes.

In a frying pan or wok, stir fry the garlic in olive oil. Then, add in all other ingredients (except green onions) and continue to stir until the sauce thickens a little.

Add in the tofu strips, bamboo shoots, and green onion and toss. Enjoy!

Nutrition

Calories: 123kcal | Carbohydrates: 11g | Protein: 10g | Fat: 5g | Saturated Fat: 1g | Sodium: 773mg | Potassium: 112mg | Fiber: 2g | Sugar: 5g | C: 4mg | Calcium: 117mg | Iron: 2mg

Oyster Sauce Mushroom

Prep Time: 5 mins

Cook Time: 10 mins

Ingredients

- 8 ounces large button mushrooms cleaned and quartered. For smaller ones, keep whole or cut in half
- 1 Tablespoon melted butter
- 1 Tablespoon oyster sauce
- 1/4 teaspoon black pepper or to taste
- 1 Tablespoon green onion thinly sliced optional

Instructions

In a large bowl, toss the mushroom with melted butter, oyster sauce, and black pepper.

Put the mushroom in a lightly greased cake pan, ait fry the mushroom at 380F (190C) for about 6-7 minutes, stir once in between.

Garnish with some green onion to serve.

Nutrition

Calories: 80kcal | Carbohydrates: 5g | Protein: 4g | Fat: 6g | Saturated Fat: 4g | Cholesterol: 15mg | Sodium: 302mg | Potassium: 361mg | Fiber: 1g | Sugar: 2g | Vitamin C: 2mg | Iron: 1mg

Fried Okra With Sriracha Mayo

Prep Time: 5 mins

Cook Time: 10 mins

Ingredients

- 15 okra
- 1 egg beaten
- 1/2 cup Japanese panko
- 3 Tablespoon freshly chopped Thai basil
- 1/4 cup mayonnaise
- 1 Tablespoon Sriracha or to taste
- 2-3 Tablespoon Mirin

Instructions

Mix chopped basil with panko and set aside.

Line the fryer basket with lightly greased aluminum foil. Dip the okra in the egg wash, roll them in panko mix, and put them in the fryer basket without stacking. Air fry at 380F (190C) for about 8 minutes, shake the basket once in between.

In the meantime, mix the mayo, sriracha, and mirin and set aside. Serve the fried okra with sriracha mayo when done.

Nutrition

Calories:337kcal | Carbohydrates: 25g | Protein: 7g | Fat: 24g | Saturated Fat: 4g | Cholesterol: 94mg | Sodium: 627mg | Potassium: 329mg | Fiber: 4g | Sugar: 7g | Vitamin C: 26mg | Calcium: 119mg | Iron: 2mg

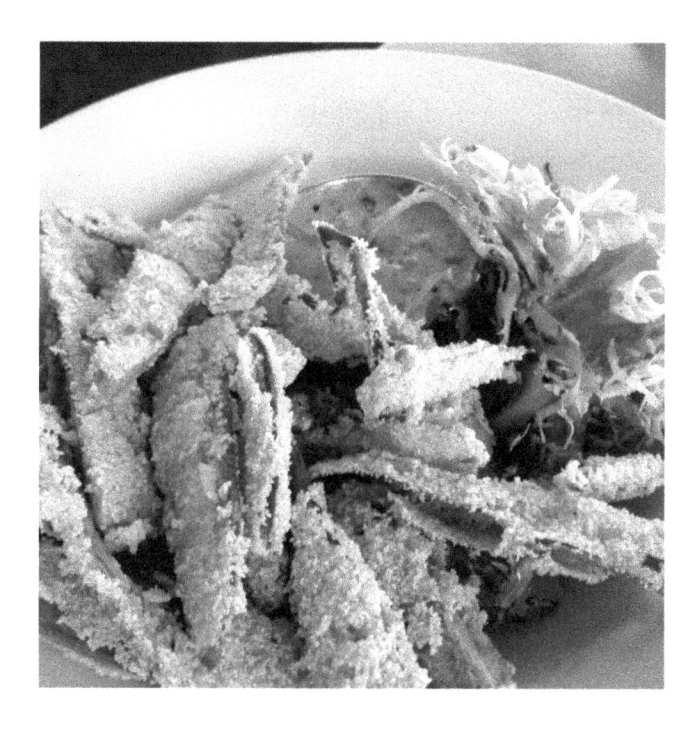

Miso Tofu

Prep Time: 10 mins

Cook Time: 20 mins

Ingredients

- 1 box firm tofu
- 2 tablespoon miso paste
- 1 teaspoon Sriracha Hot Sauce optional
- 4 teaspoon brown sugar
- 2 teaspoon sesame oil
- 2 teaspoon soy sauce
- 1 green onion thinly sliced
- 1 Tablespoon sesame seeds

Instructions

Place a kitchen towel on the counter and place the tofu on top. Put a heavy item, such as a small pot, on top of the tofu for one hour to squeeze out excess water.

In the meantime, prepare the sauce by mixing miso, Sriracha, brown sugar, sesame oil, and soy sauce. Cut tofu into 1/2-3/4 inches thick slices then cut the surface of the tofu in a crisscrossed fashion without cutting through.

Carefully put the tofu pieces into the parchment-lined fryer basket. Brush a thick layer of sauce onto the tofu and lightly dab the surface so the sauce can get into the crevices. Air fry at 400F (200C) for 10-12 minutes, brushing a layer of the sauce every 3-4 minutes until the sauce is caramelized.

Sprinkle some green onion and sesame seeds to serve.

Nutrition

Calories: 147kcal | Carbohydrates: 9g | Protein: 11g | Fat: 8g | Saturated Fat: 1g | Sodium: 517mg | Potassium: 27mg | Fiber: 2g | Sugar: 5g |Vitamin C: 1mg | Calcium: 151mg | Iron: 2mg

Maple Walnut Biscotti

Prep Time: 10 mins

Cook Time: 40 mins

Ingredients

- 1 cup all-purpose flour
- 1/3 cup packed brown sugar
- 1 1/4 teaspoons baking powder
- 1/4 teaspoon salt
- 1 egg
- 2 Tablespoon maple syrup
- 2 Tablespoon melted unsalted butter
- 1 cups coarsely chopped walnuts

Instructions

In a parchment-lined fryer basket, air fry the walnuts at 300F (150C) for 6 minutes.

In the meantime, take a large and bowl and mix all the dry ingredients. Then, add in the wet ingredients until everything is well combined. Finally, fold in the chopped walnuts and form the batter into a ball shape.

Place the ball-shaped dough on parchment paper and press it down with the palm of your hand to mold the dough into a rectangular shape with a thickness of about 1/2 inch. Air fry at 360F (180C) for 15 minutes.

Remove the rectangular cookie along with the parchment paper from the fryer basket and let cool for a few minutes. When cool enough to handle, cut it into 3/4 inch wide pieces.

Place all the pieces back into the fryer basket with the cut side up and air fry at 360 for about 10 minutes, flipping once in between with the other cut side facing up.

When done, carefully remove the biscotti from the fryer basket and let them cool completely on a cooling rack before serving.

Nutrition

Calories: 234kcal | Carbohydrates: 27g | Protein: 5g | Fat: 13g | Saturated Fat: 3g | Sodium: 85mg | Potassium: 175mg | Fiber: 1g | Sugar: 12g | Vitamin C: 1mg | Calcium: 60mg | Iron: 1mg

Kimchi Tofu Stir Fry

Prep Time: 5 mins

Cook Time: 10 mins

Ingredients

- 8 oz firm tofu (about 250g) cut into cubes
- 4 Tablespoon honey
- 2 Tablespoon Korean hot pepper paste Gochujang or to taste
- 2 Tablespoon soy sauce
- 1 Tablespoon oyster sauce
- 1 Tablespoon sesame oil
- 2 Tablespoon minced garlic
- 1/2 cup kimchi chopped
- 2 green onions cut into one-inch pieces
- 1 teaspoon sesame seeds

Instructions

Line the fryer basket with parchment paper and place the tofu cubes inside the basket without stacking. Spray the surface of the tofu with some oil and air fry at 400F (200C) for 10 minutes, flipping once in the middle.

In the meantime, in a saucepan, saute the minced garlic with sesame oil. Then, add honey, soy sauce, oyster sauce, and kimchi into the sauce to the pan and bring to boil, stirring frequently until the sauce thickens a bit.

When the tofu is done, toss the tofu in the sauce along with the green onion for about a minute. Sprinkle some sesame seeds over the tofu to serve.

Nutrition

Calories: 338kcal | Carbohydrates: 48g | Protein: 14g | Fat: 13g | Saturated Fat: 2g | Sodium: 1264mg | Potassium: 184mg | Fiber: 2g | Sugar: 37g | Vitamin C: 7mg | Calcium: 175mg | Iron: 3mg

Cheesy Roasted Potatoes

Prep Time: 20 mins

Cook Time: 20 mins

Ingredients

- 1 potato peeled and cubed
- 2 Tablespoon olive oil
- 1/2 teaspoon garlic powder
- 1/2 teaspoon paprika
- 1/4 teaspoon salt
- 1/2 teaspoon dried parsley flakes
- 1/3 cup shredded cheese

Instructions

Soak the potato cubes in cold water for at least 15 minutes then drained.

Combine all ingredients, except parsley flakes and cheese, and toss. Air fry, without stacking, in a lightly greased aluminum foil-lined fryer basket at 360F (180C) for 15-17 minutes. Stir a couple of times in between until the potato cubes are tender.

Pull the fryer basket out, sprinkle the parsley flakes and mix. Top the potato with cheese and push the basket into the air fryer unit for about a minute for the cheese to melt. Serve immediately.

Nutrition

Calories: 123kcal | Carbohydrates: 7g | Protein: 4g | Fat: 9g | Saturated Fat: 2g | Cholesterol: 7mg | Sodium: 210mg | Potassium: 220mg | Fiber: 1g | Sugar: 1g Vitamin C: 6mg | Calcium: 63mg | Iron: 2mg

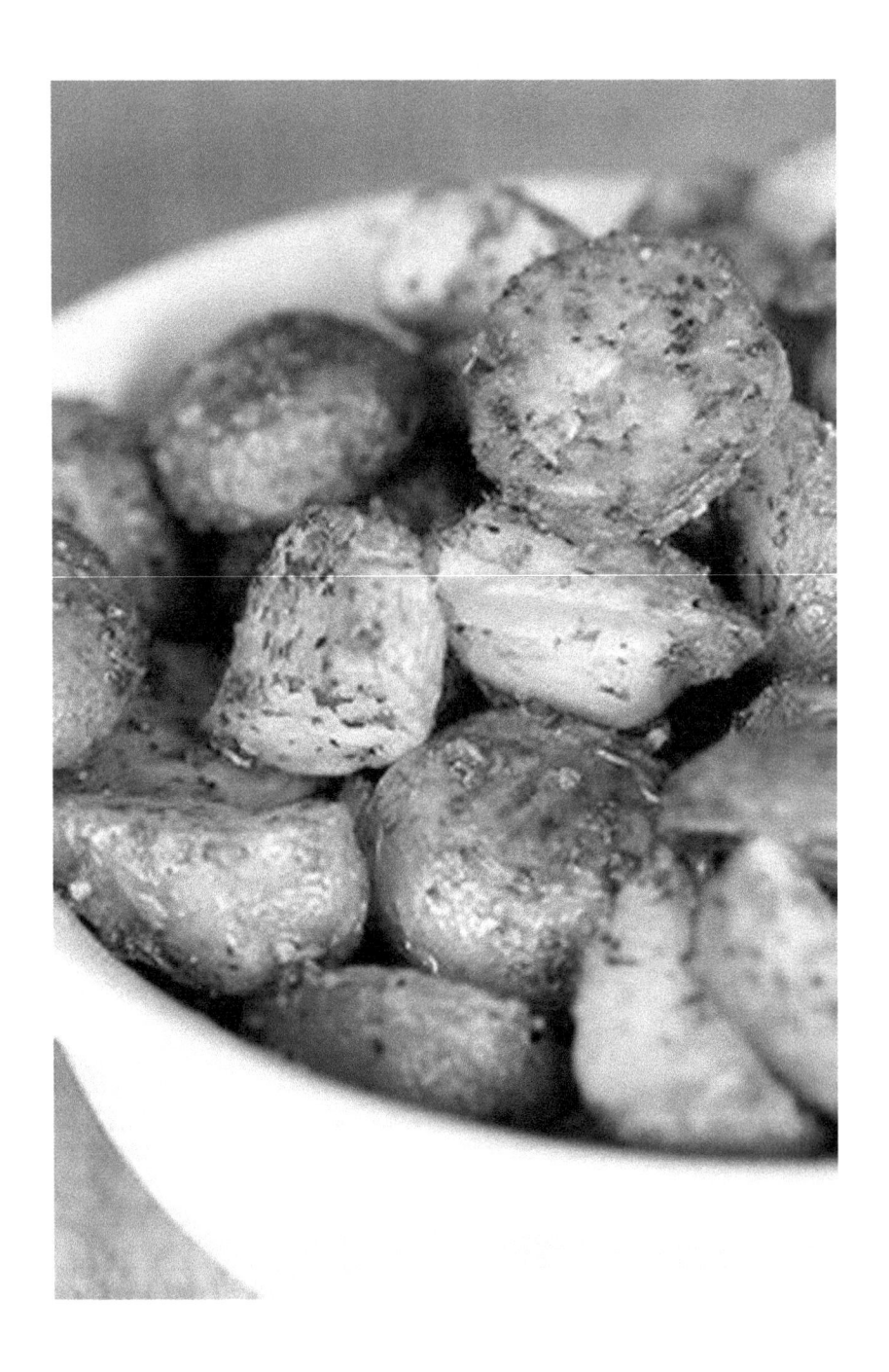

Lightning Source UK Ltd.
Milton Keynes UK
UKHW021850300421
382942UK00003B/198